Mindful Beginnings

Navigating Pregnancy with Presence and Grace

Serene Wellspring

Table of contents

Introduction

Hello, dear reader,

Pregnancy is a remarkable journey—one that encompasses not just the physical changes in your body but also a profound transformation of your mind and spirit. It's a time of anticipation, excitement, and sometimes, a touch of apprehension. As you embark on this extraordinary voyage, you may be overwhelmed with advice, stories, and well-intentioned guidance from family, friends, and the ever-enthusiastic internet.

In the midst of all this information, we invite you to take a deep breath and embark on a different kind of journey— an exploration of mindful pregnancy. This book is your trusted companion on the path to embracing the incredible experience of growing a new life within you.

Here, you won't find a list of do's and don'ts that will leave you feeling restricted or anxious. Instead, we aim to empower you with knowledge, self-awareness, and a sense of calm. We believe that the key to a mindful pregnancy lies in finding balance, in tuning in to your body's wisdom, and in nurturing not just your baby but also your own well-being.

Throughout these pages, we will delve into the physical changes, emotional rollercoasters, and practical considerations that come with pregnancy. We'll also explore mindfulness techniques that can help you navigate this incredible journey with grace and confidence.

We understand that every pregnancy is unique, and so is every mother-to-be. Whether this is your first pregnancy or your fifth, whether you're carrying one precious soul or more, whether you have a supportive partner or are going it alone, we want this book to be a source of comfort, wisdom, and inspiration.

As we embark on this journey together, remember that mindfulness isn't about perfection. It's about presence—being here, in this moment, fully embracing the beauty and complexity of pregnancy. So, let's begin this exploration of mindful pregnancy with open hearts, open minds, and a sense of wonder for the miracle unfolding within.

1

Connecting with Your Baby

The miracle of life begins with connection. Mindfulness can help you bond with your unborn child, creating a foundation for a strong, nurturing relationship.

Talk and Sing: Engage in conversations with your baby, share your thoughts, and sing lullabies or songs. Your voice is soothing and helps your baby become familiar with the sound.

Picture this: You, lounging in your favorite chair, sipping on your "pregnancy-friendly" beverage of choice (maybe it's decaf tea or sparkling water), and having a heart-to-heart with your belly. It might feel a tad strange at first, but trust us, your baby is all ears—figuratively speaking, of course!

And here's a fun tidbit: According to Partanen et al. (2013) babies actually remember and respond to the melodies they heard during pregnancy once they're born. So, don't be surprised if that lullaby you've been singing becomes your secret weapon for soothing a fussy newborn.

When you engage in conversations with your baby, sharing your thoughts, dreams, and daily anecdotes, you're doing more than just keeping yourself company, your voice becomes a source of comfort and familiarity for your little one. Your baby begins to recognize the soothing cadence of your voice, even before they can make out the words. They're tuning in to their favorite radio station— "Mom and Dad's Greatest Hits."

The Science of Soothing Sounds

Now, let's talk about singing. It's not just reserved for those who can hit high notes like a professional singer. Your baby doesn't care if you're a Grammy winner or a shower crooner. They love the sound of your voice. Singing lullabies or your favorite songs has a magical effect on your baby's developing brain (Pino et al., 2023).

As your vocal cords create those harmonious notes, the vibrations ripple through the amniotic fluid, creating a mini-concert experience for your baby. These vibrations are heard and felt by your baby, introducing them to the world of sensory stimulation. It's like hosting a private concert in the coziest concert hall ever—the womb!

The Witty Art of Conversation and Song

You might wonder, "What in the world do I talk about with a tiny human who can't talk back?" Well, pretty much anything! Think of it as your stand-up comedy routine with the world's tiniest audience.

Sure, you can discuss the weather (even if your baby has zero concept of rain or sunshine), your daily escapades (from navigating sudden food cravings to wrestling with maternity jeans), or even the latest celebrity gossip (because who doesn't want to be in the loop?).

And let's not forget the quirky side of pregnancy. You can share your baffling food cravings (pickles and ice cream, anyone?), your dramatic attempts to tie shoelaces with a burgeoning belly, and your epic battles with heartburn. Your baby might not chime in with witty comments, but you can bet they're enjoying the show!

When it comes to singing, the stage is yours. Whether you're belting out timeless lullabies or adapting the latest chart-toppers to baby-friendly versions, your baby is your biggest fan, and they're giving you a standing ovation with every kick, flutter, and wiggle.

In conclusion, talking and singing to your baby during pregnancy is not only about creating beautiful memories but also fostering a connection that will last a lifetime. So, let your voice be the lullaby that cradles your baby to sleep and the story that accompanies them on this incredible journey from the womb to your loving arms.

Gentle Touch: Place your hands on your belly and feel for movements or kicks. Gently stroking or massaging your belly can create a sense of closeness.

Ah, the exquisite art of gentle touch during pregnancy! As your belly expands and your little one's acrobatics inside become increasingly pronounced, there's a beautiful opportunity for you to engage in a sensory dialogue with your baby. We will explore the power of your touch, how it enhances your connection, and why it's not just for you but also for that tiny wonder-in-the-making.

Your Hands: Bridges to Bonding

Imagine sitting down, perhaps with a cup of soothing herbal tea (oh, the joys of caffeine-free life!), and letting your hands rest on your burgeoning belly. It's a moment of quiet contemplation, a connection that transcends words. This simple act is a bridge that links you and your baby in a comforting and profound way.

As you place your hands on your belly, you become attuned to the gentle, rhythmic movements within. It's like a secret handshake between you and your little one, your way of saying, "I'm here, and I'm listening." Your baby, in turn, responds with their own unique Morse code of kicks, rolls, and stretches, acknowledging your presence in their own silent, mysterious language.

A Symphony of Sensations

It's not just about feeling those jubilant kicks and somersaults. Your baby can sense the warmth and tenderness of your touch. As your hands caress your belly, your baby might lean into the touch, as if they're relishing a loving embrace. The amniotic fluid acts as a conductor, transmitting the sensations to your baby, creating a symphony of tactile delight.

And here's a bit of wonder: studies suggest that these early tactile experiences can enhance your baby's sense of security and emotional well-being even before they take their first breath in the outside world(Montagu, 1971). Your touch becomes the cornerstone of a foundation built on love and trust.

A Witty Ode to the Belly Rub

Rubbing your belly is an art form. It's a dance between your hands and the growing orb before you. It's a bit like polishing a crystal ball to see the future—a future filled with sleepless nights, diaper changes, and an endless supply of adorable baby onesies.

As you massage your belly, you might find yourself talking to your little inhabitant, not unlike a ship captain addressing their loyal crew. "All's well on deck, little matey!" you might jest as you feel a particularly enthusiastic kick. Your baby, in return, may provide feedback in the form of somersaults, which you could interpret as their enthusiastic approval of your belly-rubbing skills.

There's also the belly as a makeshift shelf. It's an ideal spot for balancing snacks, TV remotes, and even that elusive TV guide (if anyone still uses those). After all, multitasking is an essential skill in the journey of parenthood, and your belly makes for a convenient catch-all tray.

In conclusion, gentle touch during pregnancy is more than just a physical act. It's a language of love, a silent conversation that transcends words. So, as you rub, massage, or rest your hands on your belly, remember that you're building a bridge of connection with your baby, one touch at a time. And who knows, your baby might just be practicing their interpretive dance moves in response to your loving touch!

Mindful Bonding: Dedicate quiet moments each day to sit in stillness, close your eyes, and focus on your baby. Visualize a loving connection and send positive thoughts and emotions to your little one.

Picture this: It's a busy day, the world around you is buzzing with activity, and you have a to-do list stretching to infinity. But in the midst of it all, you take a breath, find a comfortable spot, close your eyes, and let the chaos melt away. It's a moment just for you and your baby to savor the incredible journey you're embarking on together.

These quiet interludes aren't just about calming your frazzled nerves (though that's a lovely side effect); they're an opportunity to nurture a mindful connection with your baby. As you sit in stillness, you tell your baby, "Hey there, I'm here with you now." And trust us, they can feel it.

Visualizing Love and Connection

Now, let's talk about visualization. As you close your eyes, imagine the tiny life flourishing inside you. Picture your baby in all their splendor – their tiny fingers, the delicate curve of their nose, and that little heart beating like a rhythmic drum. You're not just picturing it; you're feeling it, connecting with the essence of this new life.

As you focus on your baby, let your heart swell with love. Visualize a warm, golden light enveloping both of you, a radiant cocoon of affection and protection. These positive thoughts and emotions that you're channeling aren't just for your benefit. They're gifts to your baby, affirming your boundless love and devotion.

The Playful Side of Mindful Bonding

Have you ever tried to find a quiet spot for mindful bonding in a house filled with noisy relatives or overenthusiastic pets? It's a bit like seeking tranquility in the middle of a circus. But remember, those funny interruptions are part of your unique journey. Your baby is already learning to adapt to life's surprises.

And speaking of surprises, your baby might have some opinions during your mindful moments. You might be enjoying a serene visualization when they decide it's time for a little dance party or a soccer practice session. It's their way of saying, "I'm here, Mom, and I've got moves!"

If you find your mind wandering during these sessions, don't fret. It's all part of the mindfulness process. Gently guide your thoughts back to your baby. You're not striving for perfection; you're aiming for connection.

In conclusion, mindful bonding is a beautiful, peaceful practice that enriches your pregnancy journey. These

moments of stillness, visualizing love, and sending
positive thoughts are like love letters to your baby's heart.
So, keep those eyes closed, embrace the stillness, and let
your love flow freely to the tiny one growing within. After
all, who knows, your baby might just be enjoying these
serene moments as their own private meditation sessions!

2

Navigating Physical Changes

Your body is a remarkable vessel for new life but undergoes many changes during pregnancy. Practicing mindfulness can help you embrace these changes with grace and gratitude.

Body Scan Meditation: Start from your toes and slowly move your awareness up, acknowledging and accepting each physical change as a natural apart of the pregnancy journey.

Imagine a quiet moment, perhaps in the gentle glow of candlelight or the hush of early morning, as you embark on a body scan meditation. It's a journey that starts at your toes and gradually moves up through every inch of your body. With each step, you acknowledge and embrace the changes your body is undergoing, viewing them not as inconveniences but as natural and beautiful aspects of your pregnancy journey.

Beginning with your toes, you may notice they feel different, perhaps a bit puffier or more pampered. Moving upward, you come to your belly, where you'll find a gentle curve forming. Your skin may feel softer, your muscles adjusting to accommodate the new life within. As your awareness ascends, you'll encounter your breasts, your hips, and so many other parts of you that are subtly shifting. By the time you reach your head, you'll have traversed a landscape of transformation, leaving you with a sense of awe and reverence for the miraculous process underway.

Embracing Laughter Lines and Love Handles

Now, let's sprinkle a dash of humor into this mindful journey. Those laugh lines, once disguised with makeup, now shine like badges of honor, reminders of the joy and laughter that have enriched your life. Those love handles? They've transformed into love grips, ready to hold onto the most precious cargo of all. It's all about perspective, and what better way to embrace these changes than with a smile?

The body scan meditation isn't just about connecting with your physical self; it's also about celebrating the ever-evolving canvas on which your child's life story is being written. Your body, like an artist's brush, is creating a masterpiece. So, take a moment each day to admire your body's work in progress.

The Art of Mindful Self-Appreciation

Pregnancy is a journey of profound emotional and physical changes, a symphony of growth and transformation. It's essential to practice self-appreciation as you navigate these changes. In this chapter, we'll delve deeper into the practice of mindful self-appreciation, celebrating your body and the incredible journey it's undertaking.

A Gentle Reminder

In the hustle and bustle of daily life, we often forget the art of being gentle with ourselves. Pregnancy is a poignant opportunity to rekindle this lost art. When you catch your reflection and notice these changes, pause for a moment and offer yourself reassuring words. Remember that these shifts are a testament to the incredible journey of nurturing new life.

The truth is, you're a superhero in the making, and those "battle scars" are your badges of honor. Stretch marks, swollen feet, or fatigue are not signs of weakness but symbols of your body's remarkable adaptability. Celebrate them. They're proof of your body's unwavering commitment to your baby's well-being.

The Practice of Self-Appreciation

Now, let's get practical. How can you practice self-appreciation during pregnancy? It starts with your inner dialogue. Replace self-criticism with words of encouragement. Instead of saying, "I look so different," try saying, "I am radiant with the miracle of life."

Take breaks when you need them, and don't hesitate to ask for support. Pregnancy is a time when self-care isn't a luxury; it's a necessity. Surround yourself with people who uplift and support you, and remember, it's perfectly okay to put your feet up and enjoy some "me time."

Mindful Self-Compassion: Practice self-compassion by offering kind and reassuring words to yourself. Remind yourself that these changes are a testament to the incredible journey of nurturing new life.

Imagine a tranquil afternoon, perhaps nestled in your favorite cozy corner, as you embark on a journey of self-compassion. It's a practice that asks you to be gentle and understanding with yourself as your body undergoes these extraordinary changes. You may be wondering, "Why is this so important?" The answer is simple yet profound: it's about recognizing that these changes are a testament to the incredible journey of nurturing new life.

Embracing Your Inner Cheerleader

As you navigate the twists and turns of pregnancy, it's crucial to have your own inner cheerleader. A voice that offers kind and reassuring words when you need them the most. Instead of dwelling on perceived flaws or the inconveniences of change, remind yourself that every stretch mark, every extra pound, and every ache is a mark of your body's love and dedication to the precious life growing within.

Think of yourself as your own BFF (Best Friend Forever), ready with words of encouragement and support. Your

body is working tirelessly to create and nurture a new life
– it deserves nothing less than your utmost compassion.

Imagine talking to yourself like you would to your best
friend. If you accidentally put your shoes on the wrong
feet (blame it on pregnancy brain), would you berate your
friend or laugh it off together? You'd likely share a chuckle
and help them fix it. Extend the same kindness to yourself.

Parenthood, after all, is known for its unexpected and
humorous moments. Whether it's the unforgettable
incident involving mismatched socks or your sudden
craving for pickles and ice cream, embracing these quirks
with a sense of humor can be a delightful part of your
pregnancy experience.

A Safe Harbor for Emotions

Just like the waves of the ocean, emotions can be
unpredictable. One moment you might be overwhelmed
with joy and gratitude; the next, tears might flow for no
apparent reason. Self-compassion provides a safe harbor
for these emotional waves.

When you experience moments of doubt, fear, or sadness,
offering yourself kindness rather than self-criticism is
essential. Say to yourself, "It's okay to feel this way; I'm
human." By acknowledging and accepting your emotions
without judgment, you create a space for healing and
growth.

Self-Compassion in Action

How do you put self-compassion into action during pregnancy? Start by being mindful of your self-talk. Instead of saying, "I look so different," say, "I am beautiful, and these changes are a testament to my incredible journey." Treat yourself with the same tenderness and care you would offer a dear friend.

Remember that asking for help is an act of self-compassion. Whether it's leaning on your partner for support or seeking the advice of healthcare professionals, reaching out when you need it is an essential part of nurturing yourself during pregnancy.

Practicing body scan meditation and mindful self-compassion is a gift you give yourself during pregnancy. It's a reminder that you are strong, beautiful, and deserving of love and kindness. So, as you journey through this miraculous time, embrace the changes, offer yourself reassurance, and remember that you are creating a story of love and nurturing that will be cherished for a lifetime.

Positive Affirmations: Create positive affirmations related to your changing body. Repeat these affirmations regularly to reinforce a positive mindset. For example, "My body is beautifully designed for this journey," or "I am grateful for the changes that nourish and protect my baby." These affirmations can help you shift your perspective to one of grace and gratitude.

Imagine standing in front of the mirror, your reflection highlighting the physical changes pregnancy has brought about. In this moment, you have a choice. You can focus on perceived flaws or inconveniences, or you can choose a different path. Positive affirmations have the power to reshape your perception of self. Instead of dwelling on the aspects you wish were different, affirmations encourage you to celebrate the incredible journey your body is on. It's about shifting your focus from criticism to compassion, from doubt to appreciation.

Crafting Your Affirmations

So, how do you create these affirmations? It's simpler than you might think. Start by reflecting on your unique pregnancy journey. What aspects of your changing body do you want to celebrate and appreciate?

Perhaps it's the way your belly is gently rounding, cradling the life within. Or maybe it's the glow in your skin that speaks of the vibrant life force coursing through you. Whatever it is, let it become the centerpiece of your affirmations.

Your affirmations can be as simple or as elaborate as you like. For instance, you might repeat to yourself, "My body is beautifully designed for this journey," or "I am grateful for the changes that nourish and protect my baby." The key is to choose words that resonate with your heart.

Now take a moment to imagine, your baby decides to throw a dance party in your belly at the most unexpected moment. You might find yourself waddling like a penguin or needing assistance to tie your shoes. These quirks of pregnancy are perfect fodder for humorous affirmations.

For example, "I may waddle like a penguin, but I'm carrying precious cargo," or "I've mastered the art of asking for help, and that's a win in itself!" These affirmations not only make you smile but also remind you that the journey is filled with charming and sometimes comical moments.

The Daily Ritual of Affirmations

Positive affirmations are not just nice-sounding words; they are daily rituals that can shape your perception of self and pregnancy.

A Daily Dose of Positivity

Try starting your day with a gentle affirmation, like, "Today, I embrace the changes in my body with love and gratitude." It sets the tone for the day ahead, reminding you to celebrate your body's incredible journey.

As you repeat these affirmations, they become like daily vitamins for your mind and soul. They reinforce a positive mindset, helping you navigate the highs and lows of pregnancy with grace and resilience.

A Shield Against Negativity

Pregnancy can sometimes bring unsolicited advice or comments from well-meaning friends and family. Affirmations become your shield, deflecting negativity and self-doubt. When someone comments on your size or appearance, you can silently recite your affirmations, reminding yourself of the beauty and strength within.

Moreover, affirmations are not just for you but also for your growing baby. Your positive mindset and self-love are gifts you give to your child even before their arrival, shaping a nurturing and confident environment.

Here are some Positive Affirmations to get you started:

1. "I am creating a safe and loving environment for my baby."

2. "My body is strong and capable of nurturing new life."

3. "I trust my body's wisdom to grow and birth my baby."

4. "Each day, my baby and I grow healthier and stronger."

5. "I am connected to the divine flow of life, and it supports me."

6. "I am surrounded by love and support from my family and friends."

7. "I embrace the changes in my body as a beautiful part of this journey."

"I am prepared, both mentally and emotionally, for the arrival of my baby."

9. "I am a strong and resilient mother, capable of handling any challenge."

10. "I am filled with gratitude for the miracle of pregnancy and the gift of new life."

3

The Hormonal Tango

Pregnancy hormones can turn your emotions into a swirling dance. Mindfulness can help you find stability amidst the ups and downs of this emotional roller coaster ride.

Deep Breathing: Practice deep, slow breaths when you encounter strong emotions. Inhale deeply through your nose, allowing your belly to rise, and exhale slowly through your mouth. This simple technique can help calm your nervous system and ease intense feelings (Jallo et al., 2008).

You're standing in a checkout line, surrounded by curious glances and maybe a few judgmental eyebrows. Suddenly, you feel a surge of emotions bubbling up – frustration, irritation, or even the urge to cry because they ran out of your favorite ice cream flavor. That's when you reach for your secret weapon: deep breathing.

The technique is simple. Take a deep breath in through your nose, allowing your belly to rise like a gentle wave. Feel the air filling your lungs and your body absorbing the calming energy. Then, exhale slowly through your mouth, releasing all that tension and emotion with each breath.

Picture your belly as a helium balloon, rising gracefully with each inhalation. As you exhale, imagine all your worries and frustrations turning into bubbles, floating away like little soap bubbles at a summer picnic. It's a delightful mental image that makes deep breathing a bit more whimsical.

The Science of Serenity

Deep breathing isn't just a whimsical practice; it's firmly rooted in science. When you take those deep, slow breaths, you engage your parasympathetic nervous system, the body's natural relaxation response (Haddadi et al 2014). It's like flipping a switch from "emergency mode" to "serenity now."

The surge of oxygen with each deep breath nourishes your body and brain, promoting clarity and calmness (Jerath & Barnes, 2009). It's like giving your mind and body a refreshing sip of tranquility from the oasis of your breath.

The Power of the Breath in Everyday Life

Deep breathing is the Swiss Army knife of emotional management during pregnancy. It's there for you during morning sickness episodes when the scent of your coworker's perfume becomes your kryptonite. It's by your side during sleepless nights when your mind races with worries and to-do lists. And it's your go-to ally during those tender moments when you feel overwhelmed with love and gratitude.

You see, deep breathing doesn't discriminate. It's available anytime, anywhere, and it doesn't require special equipment or a quiet room. It's your ticket to serenity in the midst of life's joyful chaos.

The Zen of Parenting

As you practice deep breathing during pregnancy, you're also honing a valuable skill for parenthood. Parenthood, after all, is a masterclass in emotional roller coasters. When your little one decides to have a meltdown in the middle of the grocery store, you'll be equipped with your deep breathing techniques to keep your cool.

And hey, when the baby arrives, you can even introduce them to the magic of deep breaths during those restless nights. Who knows, your newborn might become a breathing guru before they even take their first steps.

Keep in mind during your pregnancy, deep breathing is your steadfast companion on this incredible journey and beyond. It's your superpower against emotional turbulence, your retreat to tranquility, and your preparation for the joys and challenges of parenthood. So, take a deep breath, embrace the serenity, and let your breath be the guiding star in your emotional galaxy.

Mindful Visualization: Close your eyes and visualize a peaceful, calming place. It could be a serene beach, a

forest, or a cozy room. Imagine yourself in that place, experiencing a sense of tranquility and emotional balance. This visualization can help you regain composure during challenging moments.

You're in the midst of a hectic day, whether it's juggling work, managing household chores, or simply dealing with the unexpected curveballs life throws your way. It's one of those moments when you feel like you're walking on a tightrope, and one wrong step might send you teetering.

This is precisely when mindful visualization comes to your rescue. You gently close your eyes and transport your mind to a serene, calming place. It could be a sun-kissed beach with waves gently lapping the shore, a quiet forest where the only sounds are the rustling leaves and chirping birds, or a cozy room where you're enveloped in warmth and comfort.

The Magic of Visualization

As you immerse yourself in this mental retreat, something incredible happens. Your body responds to your thoughts. Your breathing slows, your muscles relax, and your heart rate steadies. It's like stepping into a cocoon of tranquility in the midst of life's tempest.

You see, visualization is not just a mental exercise; it's a physical one too. By visualizing a calm and peaceful place, you're signaling to your body that it's time to unwind and find balance (Jerath & Barnes, 2009). It's your way of saying, "I've got this."

Imagine you're in the middle of a prenatal yoga class, attempting a pose that seems more like an acrobatic feat. Your balance is wavering, your patience is wearing thin, and you're contemplating whether it's time to start a new career as a contortionist.

This is the perfect moment to put your mindful visualization skills to use. Picture yourself in a yoga studio on a mountaintop, where even the wobbles are part of the graceful dance. You're not just doing yoga; you're starring in your own comedy show. The laughter that bubbles up is a reminder that, in the grand scheme of things, a wobbly yoga pose is just a blip on the radar.

Finding Peace in the Chaos

Life is a marathon, and pregnancy sometimes adds hurdles along the way. In these moments of chaos, mindful visualization is your pause button. It allows you to step back, take a deep breath, and recalibrate.

Whether you're facing a challenging conversation, managing a stressful situation, or simply needing a mental break, this visualization practice offers you a moment to regain composure. It's like a mini-vacation for your mind and soul.

Nurturing Emotional Balance

As you visualize yourself in your calming sanctuary, you're reminded of your inner strength and resilience. It's a subtle but powerful way to nurture emotional stability during pregnancy. When the storm of emotions threatens to overwhelm you, you have a safe harbor to return to, even if it exists solely in your mind.

Similar to deep breathing, mindful visualization is your portable oasis of calm during the whirlwind of pregnancy. It's your sanctuary, your reset button, and your emotional anchor. So, close your eyes, transport yourself to a place of tranquility, and remember that even in the stormiest moments, you have the power to find peace and regain composure.

4

Mindful Stress Management

As you prepare for the arrival of your baby, stress can become a companion. There are many mindfulness exercises to manage stress.

Mindful Walking: Go for a leisurely walk in a peaceful environment, such as a park or a nature trail. Pay close attention to each step you take. Feel the ground beneath your feet, notice the sensation of your muscles moving, and be aware of the sights, sounds, and smells around you. Walking mindfully can help you clear your mind, reduce stress, and connect with the present moment.

Close your eyes for a moment and picture this: You're in a tranquil environment, perhaps a lush park or a serene nature trail. The sun's warm embrace kisses your skin, and a gentle breeze plays with your hair. You embark on a leisurely walk, your surroundings a symphony of sights, sounds, and scents.

But here's the twist: You're not just strolling aimlessly; you're walking mindfully. Each step is a deliberate act, a moment of mindfulness. As your foot meets the ground, you notice the sensation beneath your sole. You're aware of the subtle shift in your muscles as they move. And your senses are engaged, taking in the world around you—the birds singing, the leaves rustling, the earthy scent of the forest.

Now, imagine you're on your mindful walk, and suddenly, you encounter a tiny critter that seems to be on a mission to outpace you. It might be a curious squirrel or a determined snail—the exact details don't matter.

What's important is that this little fellow becomes your mindfulness mascot. As you walk, you're not just focused on your own steps but also cheering on your critter friend, secretly hoping it reaches its destination. This playful visualization adds a touch of whimsy to your mindful walking experience and reminds you that mindfulness can be fun.

The Path to Clarity and Calm

The mind, during pregnancy, can be a lively carnival of thoughts, worries, and to-do lists. Mindful walking becomes your pause button. It's a moment when you step away from the noise of your thoughts and into the serenity of the present moment.

As you focus on each step, your mind naturally quiets down. Worries about the future and regrets from the past take a backseat. You become fully present in the here and now. It's like clearing the clutter from your mental workspace and creating space for calm.

Stress Reduction, One Step at a Time

Pregnancy, while beautiful, can also be demanding. From doctor's appointments to nursery preparations, the stress can add up. Mindful walking is an antidote to stress.

Studies have shown that mindful walking can reduce stress hormones in the body (Price et al., 2012). As you immerse yourself in the sensations of each step, you're offering yourself a break from the stressors of daily life. It's like a mini-retreat, a brief escape that leaves you feeling refreshed and rejuvenated.

It's a practice that connects you to your body, calms your mind, and reduces stress. So, find a peaceful environment, lace up those comfortable shoes, and let each step become a step towards serenity on this remarkable journey.

Gratitude Journaling: Keep a gratitude journal where you write down three things you're grateful for every day. These can be small moments, like feeling your baby kick, receiving support from a loved one, or experiencing a moment of peace. Reflecting on the positive aspects of your life can shift your focus away from stressors.

Imagine you're sitting in your favorite cozy corner, pen in hand and a blank journal before you. You begin by reflecting on your day, searching for three things you're grateful for. These moments can be as small or large as

getting to work on time, receiving a warm hug from a
loved one, or simply savoring a moment of peace.

As you write them down, you're not just documenting
moments but celebrating them. Gratitude journaling is like
shining a spotlight on the bright spots in your life, no
matter how seemingly insignificant they may be.

As you're journaling one evening, your baby decides to
give you an unexpected dance performance in your belly.
It's like an impromptu rave party in there, complete with
neon lights and glow sticks (at least it feels that way).

You jot down this joyful moment and add a playful note:
"Baby has impeccable timing for dance parties!" This touch
of humor not only lightens the mood but also reminds you
that even in the midst of pregnancy's quirks, there's
always something to be grateful for.

A Daily Dose of Positivity

Pregnancy, like any journey, has its share of challenges
and uncertainties. Gratitude journaling becomes your
daily touchpoint for positivity and emotional well-being.

The mind, during pregnancy, can sometimes gravitate
toward worries and stressors. Gratitude journaling is your
tool for shifting that focus. Instead of dwelling on what's
challenging, you're highlighting what's uplifting.

As you regularly jot down moments of gratitude, you train
your mind to notice the positives. It's like tuning your

mental radio to a station that plays your favorite uplifting songs. You become more attuned to the beauty and joy that surround you.

Enhancing Emotional Well-being

When you reflect on the positive aspects of your life, even on the challenging days, you're nurturing a sense of contentment and resilience. It's like building an emotional toolbox that helps you weather the ups and downs with grace.

During pregnancy, gratitude journaling is your daily ritual of celebrating the bright moments of pregnancy. It's a practice that shifts your focus toward positivity, enhances your emotional well-being, and helps you find joy in even the smallest of moments. So, pick up that pen, open your journal, and let gratitude become your daily companion on this remarkable journey.

Loving-Kindness Meditation: Practice loving-kindness meditation to cultivate feelings of love and compassion for yourself and your baby. Find a quiet space, close your eyes, and repeat phrases like "May I and my baby be happy," "May I and my baby be healthy," and "May I and my baby be safe." Extend these wishes to others as well. This meditation can promote emotional resilience and a sense of connection during pregnancy (Fredrickson et al., 2008).

Imagine this: You're in a quiet, cozy space. You close your eyes and take a deep breath, allowing the cares of the day to fall away. In this serene moment, you begin to silently repeat phrases like "May I and my baby be happy," "May I and my baby be healthy," and "May I and my baby be safe."

As you utter these gentle wishes, you're not just reciting words; you're creating a cocoon of love and compassion around yourself and your baby. Loving-kindness meditation is like wrapping your heart in a warm embrace, nurturing feelings of well-being and connection.

Now, let's picture yourself in the midst of your meditation, reciting these loving-kindness phrases with utmost sincerity when suddenly, your baby decides to give you a little "kick" of affirmation. It's like a playful nudge from your little one, a reminder that they're right there with you in this moment of connection.

You smile, and in your meditation, you add a loving, "Thank you for the encouragement, little one." This touch of humor not only lightens the mood but also reinforces the sense of togetherness that loving-kindness meditation can bring.

Cultivating Love and Resilience

Pregnancy, while filled with joy, can also come with its share of emotional twists and turns. Loving-kindness meditation becomes your compass for navigating these moments with love, compassion, and resilience.

As you delve into the practice of loving-kindness meditation, something beautiful happens. You're not just extending these wishes to yourself and your baby; you're also offering them to others. It's like sending ripples of love and kindness out into the world.

Studies have shown that loving-kindness meditation can enhance emotional resilience (Fredrickson et al., 2008). When faced with challenges or emotional ups and downs, you have a wellspring of compassion to draw upon. It's like having an emotional shield that helps you weather the storms of pregnancy with grace and inner strength.

A Tapestry of Connection

Pregnancy is not just a journey of physical changes; it's also a journey of connection. Loving-kindness meditation fosters this sense of connection, not only to your baby but to the world around you.

As you extend your wishes of happiness, health, and safety to others, you're weaving a tapestry of connection. You're acknowledging the shared human experience and the interconnections of all beings. It's like recognizing that you're part of a grand symphony, contributing your unique notes of love and kindness.

In conclusion, loving-kindness meditation is your daily ritual of love and connection during pregnancy. It's a practice that nurtures your heart, fosters emotional resilience, and reminds you of the beautiful tapestry of connection that surrounds you. Find your quiet space, close your eyes, and let the gentle phrases of loving-kindness meditation become a source of love and strength on this remarkable journey.

5

Mindful Breathing Techniques

Mindful breathing techniques can provide calm and connection during pregnancy.

Deep Belly Breathing: This simple exercise involves taking slow, deep breaths, with a focus on expanding your diaphragm and belly. Inhale deeply through your nose, allowing your belly to rise, and then exhale slowly through your mouth, letting your belly fall. Deep belly breathing calms your nervous system, reduces stress, and increases the flow of oxygen to both you and your baby (Jerath & Barnes, 2009).

Deep belly breathing—a practice you've encountered previously in this book, and now, we revisit it. It's like finding a cozy nook in your favorite bookstore, familiar yet brimming with new stories.

The Symphony of Deep Breaths

Imagine this: You're seated in a comfortable position, perhaps with your legs crossed or reclined in a chair. One hand rests gently on your chest, and the other cradles your belly. You close your eyes and initiate a slow, deliberate inhale through your nose.

As you breathe in, your diaphragm expands, and your belly rises like a gentle tide. It's a rhythmic dance, a beautiful symphony of breath and movement. Then, as you exhale, you release your breath through your mouth, and your belly falls back to its natural position. It's a gentle ebb and flow, a reminder of the miracle of breath. You and Your baby are calm. Or you are calm and your baby is taking this time to show you their new dance moves.

A Unique Connection: You and Your Baby

During pregnancy, your body undergoes remarkable changes to nurture and protect the life growing within you. Deep belly breathing becomes more than just a relaxation exercise; it's a way to connect with your baby on a profound level.

As you inhale deeply, you're not just replenishing your own oxygen supply; you're also increasing the flow of oxygen to your baby. Imagine your breath as a conduit of life, nourishing both you and your little one. It's a reminder that you're intricately connected, sharing the same breath, the same journey.

A Calm Haven Amidst Hormonal Storms

Pregnancy hormones are like the conductors of a symphony, sometimes leading to moments of crescendo and other times to soothing lullabies. Deep belly breathing serves as your calming refuge amidst these hormonal storms.

According to Jerath and Barnes (2009), deep belly breathing calms the nervous system, reducing the production of stress hormones. When you engage in this practice regularly, you're creating a sanctuary of calm for both you and your baby. It's like placing a shield of serenity around you, ensuring that moments of peace are always within reach.

Enhancing Physical and Emotional Well-being

Pregnancy often involves physical discomforts and emotional fluctuations. Deep belly breathing becomes your ally in promoting overall well-being.

As you inhale deeply, you're not just filling your lungs with air; you're also acknowledging the strength and adaptability of your body. Your diaphragm expands, your belly rises, and you're reminded of the incredible journey you're on. It's like a loving pat on your own back, a gesture of appreciation for your body's resilience.

Box Breathing: Box breathing involves inhaling for a count of 4, holding for 4, exhaling for 4, and pausing for 4 before repeating the cycle. This method can promote balance, reduce tension, and increase mindfulness, benefitting both you and your baby.

Imagine you're in a serene corner of your home, or perhaps you've found a moment of peace in a bustling park. You sit or lie down comfortably and close your eyes. As you begin, you inhale gently for a count of 4, like a soft breeze filling your lungs. It's a rhythmic dance of breath and intention.

You hold that breath for a count of 4, savoring a moment of stillness. It's like pressing the pause button on life's demands. Then, you exhale slowly for 4, releasing tension and stress with each breath. It's a gentle cascade of relaxation. Finally, you pause for 4, letting the serenity of the moment linger before starting the cycle again.

When you're in the midst of your box breathing practice, inhaling tranquility for a count of 4, when suddenly, you feel a playful flutter from your baby. It's that reminder, like a little wink from your tiny companion, reminding you that you're not alone in this journey and also reinforces the beautiful connection you share with your baby through this practice.

Finding Balance in the Whirlwind

Pregnancy, while a time of immense joy, can also bring its share of emotional whirlwinds and physical demands. Box breathing is another mindful exercise that becomes your sanctuary, offering balance, and reducing tension.

A Balancing Act

This technique promotes balance by calming your nervous system. As you inhale, hold, exhale, and pause in a rhythmic cycle, your body and mind synchronize with a sense of harmony. It's like orchestrating a beautiful symphony, where each breath is a note, and you're the conductor.

Reducing Tension, Nurturing Mindfulness

Pregnancy, as miraculous as it is, can also lead to physical discomfort and emotional tension. Box breathing is your tool for reducing tension and nurturing mindfulness.

With each exhale, you release physical tension from your body, like letting go of a bundle of balloons. As you pause, you embrace mindfulness, savoring the present moment. It's like creating a tranquil sanctuary within yourself, where both you and your baby can find solace.

Guided Imagery Breathing: Combine deep breathing with guided imagery by visualizing a peaceful and serene place, such as a beach, forest, or garden. As you inhale, imagine yourself breathing in calm and positivity from this environment, and as you exhale, release any tension or worry. This exercise enhances relaxation, reduces stress, and fosters a sense of well-being for both you and your baby.

Now imagine you're nestled in your cozy nook, eyes gently closed, and you start with a deep, peaceful inhale. As you breathe in, you conjure an image of the most serene place in your mind. It might be a sun-kissed beach, a lush forest, or a vibrant garden. You inhale, drawing in the calm and positivity that emanates from this environment.

Then, as you exhale, you release any tension, worry, or stress that may have taken up residence within you. It's like breathing out the unwanted guests, making room for serenity and well-being. It's a dance of breath and imagination.

Now, Imagine you're in the midst of your guided imagery breathing, visualizing a peaceful beach where the waves gently lap at your toes. Suddenly, in your mental oasis, you feel that reminder from your baby. That you're not alone in this serene adventure.

You chuckle and continue your practice, adding a loving thought: "Baby's joining us for a beachside meditation!" This will reinforce the special connection you share with your baby through this practice.

A Journey to Inner Peace

Pregnancy, with its myriad emotions and physical changes, can sometimes feel like a whirlwind. Guided imagery breathing becomes your sanctuary, a passport to inner peace. As you visualize your serene place and pair it with deep breathing, you're signaling to your body and mind that it's time to unwind. It's like whispering to your inner worries, "I see you, but we're choosing serenity today."

Fostering Well-being for You and Baby

The well-being of both you and your baby is of utmost importance during pregnancy. Guided imagery breathing nurtures this sense of well-being.

As you inhale, you're not just drawing in the calming energy of your serene place; you're also offering it to your baby. Your breath becomes a conduit of positivity and tranquility, enveloping both of you in a cocoon of well-being. It's like sending love letters to your baby's heart, affirming that you're on this journey together.

6

Mindful Movement

Gentle yoga and mindful movement practices tailored for pregnancy can enhance your physical and emotional well-being.

Remember to consult with your healthcare provider before beginning any new exercise routine during pregnancy. It's important to choose movements that align with your individual needs and preferences, and to prioritize safety and comfort for both you and your baby.

Prenatal Yoga: Prenatal yoga classes are designed specifically for expectant mothers, offering a gentle and supportive way to build strength, flexibility, and balance. These classes often include mindfulness and deep breathing techniques to promote relaxation and connection with your baby (Chuntharapat et al., 2008).

Prenatal yoga is your moment to embrace your changing body. It's like a gentle waltz with your own physicality, nurturing strength, flexibility, and balance. Each pose is a reminder of the incredible journey you're on.

Imagine you're in the midst of a prenatal yoga class, gracefully transitioning from one pose to another when suddenly, your baby decides to add their own twist to the routine because, they need to let you know they are right there with you. It's like having a playful yoga buddy right in your belly.

You share a knowing smile with the other moms, acknowledging that your baby is already an expert yogi. This also reinforces the connection between you and your baby during these classes.

Mindful Movement and Strength

Prenatal yoga is not just about physical postures; it's about mindful movement. It's like a journey within, a chance to connect with the wisdom of your body.

These classes often include mindfulness techniques, encouraging you to be fully present in each pose. As you move, stretch, and breathe, you're cultivating strength and flexibility while nurturing a deep connection with your baby. It's like you're writing a love letter to your little one with each yoga pose, reminding them of your bond.

Relaxation and Connection

Pregnancy can bring moments of both excitement and anxiety. Prenatal yoga becomes your tool for relaxation and connection.

Deep breathing techniques go hand in hand with prenatal yoga and are often integrated into the class. This will also help calm your nervous system and reduce stress (Beddoe et al., 2009). As you inhale, you're drawing in positive energy and sending it to your baby, nurturing a sense of connection and serenity. It's like you're weaving a tapestry of relaxation and love, enveloping both you and your baby in its warm embrace.

Prenatal yoga helps you on your journey to balance and connection during pregnancy. It's a practice that nurtures physical resilience, enhances flexibility, and deepens the bond with your baby. So, whether you're in a serene studio or practicing at home, embrace each pose, inhale serenity, and let prenatal yoga be your gentle guide on this beautiful journey.

Yoga Tips for Expectant Mothers

1. **Consult Your Healthcare Provider:** Before starting or continuing any exercise routine during pregnancy, it's essential to consult your healthcare provider. They can provide personalized guidance based on your unique circumstances.

2. **Choose Prenatal Yoga Classes:** Seek out classes specifically designed for pregnant women. These classes are tailored to your needs and often include modifications for different stages of pregnancy.

3. **Listen to Your Body:** Your body is your best guide. If a pose feels uncomfortable or causes strain, modify it or skip it. Pay attention to any pain, dizziness, or

shortness of breath and communicate with your
instructor.

4. **Stay Hydrated:** Drink water before, during, and after
   your practice to stay hydrated. Dehydration can lead
   to dizziness and discomfort.

5. **Support Your Bump:** Use props like blocks and
   cushions to support your growing belly during poses.
   This helps maintain balance and comfort.

Simple Prenatal Yoga Poses

Here are a few gentle yoga poses that can be beneficial for
expectant mothers:

1. **Mountain Pose (Tadasana):** Stand tall with feet hip-
   width apart, hands by your sides. This pose promotes
   balance and posture.

2. **Cat-Cow Stretch:** Get on your hands and knees, arch
   your back upward like a cat, then drop your belly and
   lift your head for the cow pose. This gentle flow helps
   alleviate back pain and promotes flexibility in the
   spine.

3. **Child's Pose (Balasana):** Kneel on the floor, sit back
   on your heels, and reach your arms forward. This
   relaxing pose stretches the back and provides a sense
   of calm.

4.

Warrior II (Virabhadrasana II): Stand with one foot forward and the other foot back, arms extended parallel to the floor. This pose strengthens the legs and helps maintain balance.

5. **Butterfly Pose (Baddha Konasana):** Sit with your feet together, knees bent outward. Gently press your knees toward the floor. This pose stretches the groin and can ease discomfort in the pelvis.

6. **Savasana (Corpse Pose):** Lie on your left side with a pillow between your knees to support your hips. This position promotes relaxation and can relieve pressure on the lower back.

Remember, the goal of prenatal yoga is not to push your limits but to nurture your body and connect with your baby. Each pose and breath should be a source of comfort and serenity. With the right guidance and awareness, prenatal yoga can be a beautiful addition to your journey of pregnancy.

Pilates for Pregnancy: Prenatal Pilates focuses on strengthening the core, improving posture, and enhancing overall body awareness. It's a low-impact exercise option that can help alleviate back pain and discomfort while encouraging mindfulness of movement and breath.

Prenatal Pilates is your gateway to core strength, and it begins with a deep inhale and a gentle exhale. This practice emphasizes the core muscles, not just the visible abdominal muscles but also the deeper ones that support your spine. It's like weaving a protective cocoon around your center, nurturing both your body and your baby.

Before we dive deeper, your little bean inside would like to remind you that you are not alone. Picture yourself in a prenatal Pilates class, engaged in a core-strengthening exercise when, suddenly, you feel a playful "tumble" from your baby. It's like your little one's way of saying, "I'm working on my core too!"

You share a knowing smile with the other moms, appreciating the shared journey of strength and resilience, both inside and out.

Strength, Posture, and Comfort

Prenatal Pilates can help serve as your foundation for physical resilience and comfort during pregnancy. The focus on core strength helps alleviate back pain and discomfort, common companions of expectant mothers (Güder, 2018).

As you engage in controlled movements, you're not just building strength; you're also improving posture. It's like writing love letters to your spine, ensuring it stands tall and supports you throughout your journey.

Mindfulness in Motion

Prenatal Pilates encourages mindfulness in motion. Each movement is intentional, each breath is deliberate. You become aware of the connection between your body, your breath, and your baby. It's like a dance of harmony, where each step is a celebration of the beautiful journey you're on.

Prenatal Pilates can be your key to strength and mindfulness during pregnancy. It's a practice that nurtures your core, improves posture, and fosters a mindful connection between you and your baby. So, embrace each movement, inhale strength, and let prenatal Pilates be another gentle guide on this magnificent journey.

Pilates Tips for Expecting Mothers

1. **Consult Your Healthcare Provider:** Always consult your healthcare provider before starting any new exercise routine during pregnancy. They can provide tailored guidance based on your individual needs and any potential medical concerns.

2. **Choose Prenatal Pilates Classes:** Seek out classes or instructors who specialize in prenatal Pilates. These classes are designed with your safety and comfort in mind, offering modified exercises suitable for each stage of pregnancy.

3. **Mindful Warm-Up:** Begin your practice with a gentle warm-up to prepare your body for movement. This could include gentle stretching and deep breathing to connect with your body and baby.

4. **Focus on Alignment:** During your practice, pay close attention to your body's alignment. Maintain a

neutral spine position, avoiding any movements that strain your back or pelvis.

Simple Prenatal Pilates Exercises

Here are a few gentle Pilates exercises that can be beneficial for expectant mothers:

1. **Pelvic Tilts:** Lie on your back with your knees bent and feet flat on the floor. Inhale to prepare, then exhale as you tilt your pelvis gently upward, engaging your core. Inhale to release. This exercise helps strengthen your pelvic muscles and lower back.

2. **Leg Circles:** Lie on your back with your legs extended upward. Circle your legs gently, inhaling as you bring them down and exhaling as you lift them back up. This exercise promotes hip mobility and strengthens your abdominal muscles.

3. **Bird Dog (Quadruped):** Begin on your hands and knees, with wrists aligned under shoulders and knees under hips. Extend your right arm forward and your left leg backward, keeping your back straight. Inhale, and as you exhale, bring your elbow and knee toward each other, rounding your back. Inhale to extend again. This exercise enhances balance and stability.

4. **Squats:** Stand with your feet shoulder-width apart. Inhale as you bend your knees and lower your body into a squat position. Exhale as you return to the

starting position. This exercise strengthens your leg muscles and supports a healthy posture.

5. **Kegels:** Sit or lie down comfortably. Imagine you're trying to stop the flow of urine, contracting your pelvic floor muscles. Hold for a few seconds, then release. Repeat this exercise to strengthen your pelvic floor, which can be especially beneficial during pregnancy and postpartum.

Remember that the goal of prenatal Pilates is to nurture your body and connect with your baby. Each exercise should be performed with awareness and comfort, and you should never push yourself to the point of discomfort. With these simple exercises and mindful guidance, prenatal Pilates can be a wonderful addition to your pregnancy journey.

Swimming: Swimming and water aerobics are excellent options for pregnant women. The buoyancy of the water reduces the impact on joints, providing relief from common pregnancy discomforts (Sibley et al., 1981). **Mindful laps or gentle water movements can promote relaxation and reduce stress.**

Picture yourself at a tranquil pool, the water glistening under the gentle sun. As you step into the pool, you feel the buoyancy of the water cradle your body, and it's like a warm embrace from nature herself. Swimming is your gateway to relief, and it begins with the simplest of strokes.

The buoyancy of the water is a gift to your joints, reducing the impact and offering sweet relief from the weight of pregnancy. It's like a gentle massage for your entire body, a moment of weightlessness that allows you to glide effortlessly.

Imagine yourself in the pool, gracefully swimming your mindful laps, when suddenly, you feel a playful "nudge" from your baby. They're saying, "I'm here, enjoying the water too!"

You chuckle and continue your aquatic adventure, savoring the connection you share with your baby, even in the depths of the pool.

Relief from Common Discomforts

Mindful laps or gentle water movements encourage you to be fully present in the moment. As you move through the water, the rhythmic sound of your breath becomes a soothing mantra. It's like a dance of serenity, where each movement brings you closer to inner peace.

Swimming and water aerobics are your aquatic allies during pregnancy. They offer relief from common discomforts, promote relaxation, and reduce stress. Whether you're gliding through a serene pool or participating in water aerobics with fellow moms, embrace the water's embrace, inhale tranquility, and let swimming be your gentle guide on this watery adventure of motherhood.

Swimming Tips for Expectant Mothers:

1. **Consult Your Healthcare Provider:** Before starting or continuing any exercise routine during pregnancy, including swimming, consult your healthcare provider. They can provide personalized guidance based on your health and any specific pregnancy-related concerns.

2. **Choose a Suitable Environment:** Seek out swimming pools that are well-maintained and properly chlorinated to ensure water hygiene. Public or private pools with lifeguards on duty can offer an extra layer of safety and peace of mind.

3. **Select Comfortable Swimwear:** Invest in comfortable and supportive swimwear designed for pregnant women. Maternity swimsuits are designed to accommodate your growing belly and provide adequate support.

4. **Stay Hydrated:** While swimming, it's easy to forget about hydration. Bring a water bottle to the pool area and take breaks to drink water to stay properly hydrated.

5. **Warm-Up and Cool Down:** Just like any exercise, it's important to warm up and cool down. Spend a few minutes walking in the water or doing gentle stretches before and after your swim to prepare your body.

Simple Swimming and Water Aerobics Exercises

Here are a few simple exercises suitable for expectant mothers in the pool:

1. **Water Walking:** Stand in chest-deep water and walk forward and backward. The water's resistance adds a gentle workout for your legs and core.

2. **Leg Lifts:** Hold onto the pool's edge or use a floating device for support. Lift one leg at a time to the side, front, and back. This exercise strengthens your leg muscles and helps maintain balance.

3. **Water Cycling:** Hold onto the edge of the pool, and simulate cycling motions with your legs. This gentle exercise is excellent for leg and hip flexibility.

4. **Floating Relaxation:** Allow yourself a few moments to simply float on your back, enjoying the weightlessness and relaxation the water provides. Close your eyes, take deep breaths, and savor the serenity.

5. **Water Aerobics:** Consider joining a water aerobics class designed for expectant mothers. These classes are led by instructors who specialize in prenatal fitness and can guide you through safe and effective exercises.

Remember, the key to an enjoyable and beneficial swimming experience during pregnancy is to listen to your body. If you feel any discomfort, fatigue, or dizziness, it's essential to take a break and rest. Swimming and water aerobics offer a wonderful opportunity to stay active, relieve discomfort, and connect with your body and baby, all within the soothing embrace of the water.

Prenatal Dance: Some dance classes, specifically designed for pregnant women, offer a fun and expressive way to stay active. Dance can help improve circulation, balance, and mood while allowing you to connect with your body and your baby through movement (Sanders, 2008).

Imagine you're in a room filled with fellow expectant mothers, each with a unique glow and story. The room is alive with the sounds of laughter and rhythmic beats, and you find yourself swaying to the music. Prenatal dance is your ticket to freedom, and it begins with a simple step.

Prenatal dance classes are carefully designed to be safe and enjoyable during pregnancy. They offer a space where you can connect with your inner dancer while embracing the beautiful changes your body is going through. It's like a vibrant celebration of life itself.

Cultivating Vitality and Connection

Pregnancy is a journey of vitality and connection, and prenatal dance becomes your lively companion, enhancing circulation, balance, and mood.

As you sway, twirl, and move to the music, you're boosting circulation throughout your body, ensuring that vital nutrients reach both you and your baby. It's like a vibrant heartbeat of life coursing through your veins.

Dancing also improves balance, which can sometimes be compromised during pregnancy due to shifting weight and changing posture. With each step, you're finding equilibrium, gracefully navigating the journey ahead.

Mood Elevation and Connection

Pregnancy can be a rollercoaster of emotions, and staying connected with your body and your baby is essential. Prenatal dance becomes your emotional anchor.

The music and movement elevate your mood, releasing endorphins and creating a sense of joy (Price et al., 2012). It's like a dance of happiness, a reminder that you're embracing the beauty of life in its purest form.

As you sway to the rhythm, you're also connecting with your baby through movement. They can feel the gentle dance, and it's like a conversation in the language of love and motion.

Dancing Tips for Expecting Mothers:

1. **Consult Your Healthcare Provider:** Before starting any new exercise routine during pregnancy, including prenatal dance, consult your healthcare provider. They can provide personalized guidance based on your health and any specific pregnancy-related concerns.

2. **Choose Prenatal Dance Classes:** Seek out dance classes specifically designed for pregnant women. These classes are tailored to your needs and offer choreography that is safe and suitable for pregnancy.

3. **Listen to Your Body:** Your body is your best guide. If a dance move feels uncomfortable or causes any discomfort, modify it or skip it. Pay attention to any fatigue or shortness of breath and communicate with your instructor.

4. **Stay Hydrated:** Dancing can be a joyful and energizing activity, but it's essential to stay hydrated. Bring a water bottle to your dance class and take sips as needed to maintain hydration.

Simple Prenatal Dance Moves

Here are a few gentle dance moves suitable for expectant mothers:

1. **Swaying Side to Side:** Stand with your feet hip-width apart and gently sway your hips from side to side. You can add arm movements to complement the sway. This move is like a gentle dance with your changing center of gravity.

2. **Circle of Love:** Stand with your feet shoulder-width apart, and slowly trace a circle with your hips. This fluid motion is like a loving embrace for your baby, and it can alleviate tension in the lower back.

Floating Arms: Extend your arms gracefully to the sides, and imagine your fingers are touching the surface of water. Slowly move your arms in fluid, circular motions. This move enhances circulation and grace.

4. **Lift and Lower:** Stand tall and gently lift one heel off the floor while pointing your toe. Lower it back down, and then switch to the other heel. This exercise strengthens the calf muscles and promotes balance.

5. **Partner Dance:** If you're taking a prenatal dance class, enjoy partner dances with your fellow moms-to-be. Holding hands or linking arms while dancing in a circle creates a sense of camaraderie and connection.

Remember, the goal of prenatal dance is not perfection but celebration. Let the music guide you, and allow your body to move with grace and joy. With the right guidance and a mindful approach, prenatal dance can be a beautiful and expressive way to connect with your body, your baby, and the rhythm of life during pregnancy.

7

Mindful Eating

Your diet impacts both you and your baby. Explore the concept of mindful eating, making choices that nourish both body and soul.

Choose Whole, Nutrient-Rich Foods: Opt for foods that are as close to their natural state as possible. Fresh fruits, vegetables, whole grains, lean proteins, and healthy fats provide essential nutrients that nourish your body and support your well-being.

Imagine you're in your kitchen, surrounded by a colorful array of fresh produce. The scent of herbs and spices fills the air, and you're about to create a vibrant salad with a rainbow of vegetables. Choosing whole, nutrient-rich foods is your gateway to vitality, and it begins with a simple bite.

Whole foods are as close to their natural state as possible. They're unprocessed, unrefined, and bursting with essential nutrients. It's like Mother Nature's gift to your body, a delicious offering of health and well-being.

Before we delve deeper, let's let your little sprout give you their reminder. Picture yourself in the grocery store, scrutinizing the labels of processed foods with an amused expression. You're like a detective on a mission to uncover the truth behind those mysterious ingredients.

As you reach for whole, nutrient-rich foods, you feel a nudge or jab to your rib. As you catch your breath, you chuckle and think maybe your little one is giving you some hidden message to head to the snack aisle after you grab the veggies.

Sustaining Health and Well-Being

Pregnancy is a time when nourishing your body takes center stage. Whole, nutrient-rich foods become your allies in sustaining health and well-being.

Fresh fruits and vegetables provide vitamins, minerals, and fiber that promote digestion and boost your immune system. Whole grains offer complex carbohydrates for sustained energy. Lean proteins are essential for fetal development, and healthy fats nourish your brain and support hormone production (Thornton et al., 2006).

Choosing whole foods is like a symphony of nutrients, each playing a crucial role in the grand performance of pregnancy. It's like a culinary symphony where each note is perfectly timed, ensuring you remain energized and vibrant throughout the day.

Ultimately, choosing whole, nutrient-rich foods is your harmonious gift to yourself and your baby during pregnancy. These foods provide essential nutrients, sustain energy, and contribute to your overall sense of well-being. So, whether you're preparing a colorful salad, enjoying a hearty bowl of oatmeal, or savoring a piece of fresh fruit, relish in the flavors of nature's bounty and let whole foods be your nourishing companions on this extraordinary journey of motherhood.

Savor the Flavor and Portions: Engage your senses by appreciating the colors, textures, and aromas of your food. Take the time to fully enjoy your meals, allowing your body to register satisfaction and contentment. Listen to your body's hunger and fullness cues, and aim to eat until you're satisfied. This helps promotes a balanced relationship with food.

Picture you're seated at the dining table, a beautifully prepared meal before you. The colors on your plate are a masterpiece, the textures a symphony of sensations, and the aromas a fragrant overture. Savoring the flavor is like an orchestra of senses, where every bite is a note in the melody of your meal.

Mindful mommas, it's time to engage your senses fully. Take a moment to appreciate the vibrant hues of your vegetables, the tantalizing textures of your grains, and the alluring aromas of your dishes. As you bring each bite to your lips, let it linger on your taste buds. It's a culinary journey, a dance of flavors that invites you to slow down and fully immerse yourself in the experience.

Before we move on, Imagine yourself in a delightful showdown with a decadent dessert. You're captivated by its appearance, your fork poised for that first irresistible bite.

It's like a playful dance between your willpower and the dessert's charm.

With a wink and a nod, you savor each bite, allowing the flavors to unfold like a well-written plot twist. It's a reminder that mindful eating is not about restriction but about relishing the joys of food with a mindful heart.

Mastering Portion Control: Listening to Your Body

As you navigate the culinary landscape, remember that portion control is your compass. It encourages you to pay heed to your body's cues of hunger and fullness, guiding you towards a harmonious relationship with food. It's like a culinary dance, where you aim to eat until you're satisfied rather than overstuffed.

Incorporate portion control into your meals by starting with smaller portions and allowing yourself to savor every bite. Listen to your body's signals—it will let you know when it's time to take another bite and when you've had enough. This practice not only supports a healthy weight but also cultivates a balanced and respectful connection with food.

Balancing Act: Satisfaction with Every Meal

Pregnancy can bring an array of cravings and dietary changes. Finding satisfaction in your meals is a vital part of the mindful eating journey.

With each bite, savor the flavors, textures, and aromas. Let your senses revel in the sensory symphony of your food. You'll naturally become more attuned to your body's signals of hunger and fullness as you engage with your meals. Let these practices guide you towards a balanced and joyful relationship with food—one that nurtures not only your body but also your soul as you embrace the incredible journey of motherhood.

Cultivate Gratitude: Before each meal, take a moment to express gratitude for the food in front of you. Recognize the effort and resources that went into producing your meal, and acknowledge the nourishment it provides. This practice fosters a sense of connection and mindfulness around eating.

You're about to enjoy a meal, the table set with care, and your senses awakened to your food's delightful aromas and colors. But before you take that first bite, you pause. You take a moment to express gratitude—for the food itself, for the hands that prepared it, and for the Earth that provided its bounty.

Cultivating gratitude is like a heartfelt prelude to your meal. It's an acknowledgment of the effort and resources that went into producing your food, a recognition of the nourishment it offers, and a celebration of the interconnectedness of all beings involved in its journey from farm to table.

You are in a playful conversation with your unborn baby. You share your gratitude for the meal you're about to enjoy, and in your mind's eye, you imagine your baby responding with a delighted kick or flutter.

It's a reminder that gratitude can be a joyful exchange, not just between you and your food but also between you and the precious life growing within you. It's a heartwarming connection that adds a touch of sweetness to your mindful eating experience.

Nourishing the Body and Soul

Gratitude deepens your connection to the food on your plate. As you express thanks, you become more aware of the flavors, textures, and aromas. You savor each bite, fully immersing yourself in the culinary moment.

This practice fosters mindfulness around eating. It reminds you to slow down and appreciate the nourishment in front of you. As you become attuned to the present, you're less likely to rush through your meals, allowing your body to digest and absorb nutrients more efficiently.

Cultivating a Joyful Dining Experience

Expressing gratitude before eating can also be a wonderful way to involve your partner or family in this mindful practice. It deepens your sense of connection with loved ones, reinforcing the bonds of togetherness.

Keep in mind, cultivating gratitude before each meal is a heartfelt practice that elevates your connection to food, nurtures mindfulness, and adds a touch of joy to your dining experience. It nourishes not only your body but also your soul as you navigate the profound journey of motherhood.

Healthy Recipe Ideas

Breakfast

Spinach and Feta Omelette

For the Omelette:

- 2 large eggs

- 2 tablespoons milk or dairy-free milk substitute (if lactose intolerant)

- 1/2 cup fresh spinach leaves, chopped

- 1/4 cup crumbled feta cheese

- Salt and pepper to taste

- 1 teaspoon olive oil for cooking

Instructions:

1. In a bowl, whisk together the eggs and milk. Season with a pinch of salt and pepper.

2.

Heat the olive oil in a non-stick skillet over medium heat.

3. Pour the egg mixture into the skillet and let it cook for a minute or two until the edges start to set.

4. Sprinkle the chopped spinach and crumbled feta cheese evenly over one half of the omelette.

5. Carefully fold the other half of the omelette over the filling using a spatula.

6. Cook for another 2-3 minutes until the omelette is fully cooked and the cheese is melted.

7. Slide the omelette onto a plate, cut it in half, and serve.

Vegan Berry Breakfast Bowl

For the Smoothie Bowl:

- 1 cup mixed berries (such as strawberries, blueberries, and raspberries)

- 1 ripe banana

- 1/2 cup almond milk (or any plant-based milk of your choice)

- 1/4 cup rolled oats

- 2 tablespoons chia seeds

- 1 tablespoon almond butter (or peanut butter)

- 1 teaspoon maple syrup (optional, for sweetness)

Toppings:

- Sliced bananas

- Fresh berries

- Chopped nuts (almonds, walnuts, or pecans)

- Coconut flakes

- A drizzle of honey or more maple syrup (optional)

Instructions:

1. In a blender, combine the mixed berries, ripe banana, almond milk, rolled oats, chia seeds, almond butter, and maple syrup (if using). Blend until smooth and creamy.

2. Pour the smoothie into a bowl.

3. Top with sliced bananas, fresh berries, chopped nuts, and coconut flakes.

If desired, drizzle a little extra honey or maple syrup
for added sweetness.

*** This recipe is inherently gluten-free as long as you use
certified gluten-free oats (some oats can be cross-
contaminated with gluten during processing). The other
ingredients are naturally gluten-free.*

Lunch

Grilled Chicken and Quinoa Salad

For the Salad:

- 4 oz grilled chicken breast, sliced

- 1 cup cooked quinoa

- 1 cup mixed greens (spinach, kale, arugula, etc.)

- 1/2 cup cherry tomatoes, halved

- 1/4 cup cucumber, diced

- 1/4 cup red bell pepper, diced

For the Dressing:

- 2 tablespoons extra-virgin olive oil

- Juice of 1 lemon

- 1 teaspoon honey (or maple syrup for a vegan option)

- Salt and pepper to taste

Instructions:

1. In a large bowl, combine the cooked quinoa, mixed greens, cherry tomatoes, cucumber, and red bell pepper.

2. Top the salad with the sliced grilled chicken.

3. In a small bowl, whisk together the olive oil, lemon juice, honey (or maple syrup), salt, and pepper to make the dressing.

4. Drizzle the dressing over the salad and toss to combine.

5. Serve the grilled chicken and quinoa salad.

Vegan Quinoa and Chickpea Salad

Lunch: Vegan Quinoa and Chickpea Salad

For the Salad:

- 1 cup cooked quinoa (cooled)

- 1 can (15 oz) chickpeas, drained and rinsed

- 1 cup cherry tomatoes, halved

- 1 cucumber, diced

- 1/2 red onion, finely chopped

- 1/4 cup fresh parsley, chopped

- 1/4 cup fresh mint leaves, chopped

For the Dressing:

- Juice of 1 lemon

- 2 tablespoons olive oil

- 1 clove garlic, minced

- Salt and pepper to taste

Instructions:

1. In a large bowl, combine the cooked quinoa, chickpeas, cherry tomatoes, cucumber, red onion, parsley, and mint.

2. In a small bowl, whisk together the lemon juice, olive oil, minced garlic, salt, and pepper to make the dressing.

Drizzle the dressing over the salad and toss to combine.

4. Serve immediately or refrigerate for later. The flavors will meld together nicely if allowed to sit for a while.

***This recipe is naturally gluten-free as long as you ensure the quinoa is not cross-contaminated with gluten during processing.*

Dinner

Baked Salmon and Roasted Vegetables

For the Salmon:

- 2 salmon fillets

- 1 tablespoon olive oil

- 1 teaspoon lemon juice

- 1 teaspoon dried herbs (such as thyme, rosemary, or dill)

- Salt and pepper to taste

For the Roasted Vegetables:

- 2 cups mixed vegetables (carrots, broccoli, zucchini, etc.), cut into bite-sized pieces

- 1 tablespoon olive oil

- 1/2 teaspoon garlic powder

- Salt and pepper to taste

Instructions:

1. Preheat your oven to 375°F (190°C).

2. In a bowl, whisk together the olive oil, lemon juice, dried herbs, salt, and pepper. Brush this mixture over the salmon fillets.

3. Place the salmon fillets on a baking sheet lined with parchment paper.

4. In a separate bowl, toss the mixed vegetables with olive oil, garlic powder, salt, and pepper.

5. Spread the seasoned vegetables on another baking sheet.

6. Bake both the salmon and vegetables in the preheated oven for about 15-20 minutes or until the salmon flakes easily with a fork and the vegetables are tender and slightly crispy.

7. Serve the baked salmon alongside the roasted vegetables.

Vegan Lentil and Vegetable Stir-Fry

For the Stir-Fry Sauce:

- 1/4 cup low-sodium soy sauce (or tamari for gluten-free)

- 2 tablespoons maple syrup

- 1 tablespoon rice vinegar

- 1 teaspoon sesame oil

- 1 teaspoon cornstarch

For the Stir-Fry:

- 1 cup dried green or brown lentils, cooked

- 2 cups mixed vegetables (bell peppers, broccoli, snap peas, carrots, etc.)

- 1 tablespoon vegetable oil (such as sesame or olive oil)

- 3 cloves garlic, minced

- 1-inch piece of ginger, minced

- Cooked brown rice or quinoa for serving

Instructions:

1. In a small bowl, whisk together all the ingredients for the stir-fry sauce. Set aside.

2. Heat the vegetable oil in a large skillet or wok over medium-high heat. Add the minced garlic and ginger and stir-fry for about 30 seconds until fragrant.

3. Add the mixed vegetables to the skillet and stir-fry for 3-5 minutes until they start to become tender.

4. Add the cooked lentils and stir to combine.

5. Pour the stir-fry sauce over the mixture and continue to stir-fry for another 2-3 minutes until the sauce thickens and coats the vegetables and lentils.

6. Serve the lentil and vegetable stir-fry over cooked brown rice or quinoa.

***The sauce in this recipe contains soy sauce, which typically contains gluten. To make this recipe gluten-free, you can use tamari (gluten-free soy sauce) instead of regular soy sauce, and ensure that all other ingredients are gluten-free.*

8

Journaling and Reflection

Keeping a pregnancy journal can be a beautiful way to track your thoughts, feelings, and the journey itself. It can also serve as a gentle reminder to cultivate gratitude and mindfulness along the way.

Daily Reflection: Set aside a few minutes each day to jot down your thoughts, feelings, and experiences. Reflect on your physical sensations, emotions, and any notable moments during your pregnancy. This daily practice encourages self-awareness and helps you stay present in the moment.

You find your cozy nook, a warm beverage by your side, and a notebook that's as eager to listen as your closest friend. Daily reflection is your daily appointment with mindfulness—a precious few minutes to pause, take stock, and put your thoughts and feelings into words. It's like a love letter to your future self, a testament to the evolving landscape of your pregnancy.

Daily reflection is your compass to self-awareness. It encourages you to explore your physical sensations, to embrace your emotions, and to capture the mosaic of your pregnancy moments. It's a gentle nudge to stay present in the whirlwind of pregnancy, reminding you to savor each moment as it unfolds.

Before we dive deeper into the beauty of daily reflection, picture yourself in a playful conversation with your journal. You might share the comical side of those pregnancy cravings, the melodrama of mood swings, or the anticipation of your little one's arrival. In your mind's eye, your journal responds with witty observations or comforting advice.

It's a reminder that daily reflection isn't just about capturing profound thoughts; it's also about embracing the delightful quirks and idiosyncrasies of pregnancy. Your journal becomes a trusted confidant, listening without judgment and occasionally sharing a chuckle.

Mindful Moments in Pregnancy

As you embark on your daily reflection, you're also embarking on a journey of mindfulness. With each word you jot down, you are anchoring yourself in the present. Mindfulness is about being fully present, and your journal becomes a bridge to that state of awareness.

Through your journaling practice, you can explore the intricate tapestry of your pregnancy journey—the sensations in your body, the emotions in your heart, and the thoughts that dance through your mind. It's like catching fireflies in a jar, capturing the fleeting but beautiful moments that make up your unique pregnancy experience.

Self-Discovery Through Reflection

Daily reflection isn't just about documenting your experiences; it's also about self-discovery. It's a mirror that reflects the evolving landscape of your inner world. As you write, you may uncover new facets of yourself, your dreams, and your aspirations as a mother.

In the quiet moments of journaling, you have the space to explore your hopes, your fears, and your dreams. It's a form of self-care that allows you to nurture your emotional well-being and build resilience as you navigate the journey of pregnancy.

Track Milestones: Use your journal to record significant milestones and events throughout your pregnancy, such as your baby's first kick, your prenatal appointments, and even your changing body measurements. This helps you appreciate the journey and creates a sense of connection with your growing baby.

Imagine your pregnancy journal as a time capsule, ready to capture the precious moments that make up your journey. Whether it's the flutter of your baby's first kick, the joy of prenatal appointments, or the fascinating changes in your body measurements, your journal becomes the keeper of these treasures. It's like preserving the fleeting magic of pregnancy, one page at a time.

The Power of Milestones

Every pregnancy is a unique journey, and every milestone is a testament to the incredible transformation happening within you. Tracking these milestones in your journal is a way of acknowledging and celebrating these moments. It's like giving your journey a voice, one that whispers stories of growth, love, and anticipation.

Each entry in your journal becomes a snapshot of your experience—a reminder of your baby's first movements, the nurturing care of your prenatal appointments, and the physical changes that manifest the miracle of life. As you revisit these milestones, you'll find yourself marveling at the profound journey you're undertaking.

Connection Through Journaling

The act of tracking milestones creates a deep connection between you and your baby. It's like a silent conversation, a way of sharing the experience of pregnancy. Through your journal, you express your love, your hopes, and your dreams for the little one growing within you. It's a bond that transcends words, an unspoken connection that weaves a tapestry of love and anticipation.

As you turn the pages of your journal, you'll discover that it's not just a record of your pregnancy; it's a testament to the enduring connection you share with your baby. It's a precious gift you can one day share with your child—a treasure trove of memories that captures the magic of this extraordinary journey.

Tracking milestones in your pregnancy journal is a way of cherishing the moments, creating a profound connection

with your growing baby, and embracing the beautiful
tapestry of pregnancy.

**Express Emotions: Your journal is a safe space to express
your feelings, whether they're joy, anxiety, excitement, or
uncertainty. Writing allows you to process and validate
these emotions, promoting emotional well-being.**

Imagine your journal as a canvas and your emotions as
the vibrant colors of a beautiful painting. Pregnancy is a
masterpiece, and every emotion you feel is a brushstroke
that adds depth and richness to your journey. Whether it's
the exhilaration of baby kicks, the occasional anxiety
about the unknown, or the sheer excitement of becoming a
mom, your journal welcomes it all.

A Splash of Humor

Before we dive into the depths of emotions, let's add a
splash of humor. Picture yourself in a playful conversation
with your journal. You might share your excitement about
baby shopping sprees or the amusement of baby name
brainstorming sessions. In your mind's eye, your journal
responds with empathetic words and perhaps a witty
comment or two.

It's a reminder that journaling isn't just about expressing
heavy emotions; it's also about celebrating the lighter,
more humorous aspects of pregnancy. Your journal
becomes your companion, listening to your stories,
offering solace when needed, and sharing a laugh when
appropriate.

Processing Through Writing

Emotions, whether they're exhilarating or challenging, are a natural part of the pregnancy experience. Writing in your journal is like offering your emotions a seat at the table. It's an act of self-compassion, a way of saying, "I see you, and I honor what you're going through." It's a gentle embrace of your feelings.

As you pour your emotions onto the pages, you'll find that writing helps you process and validate what you're experiencing. It's like sorting through a treasure chest of feelings, acknowledging their presence, and allowing them to breathe. It's a therapeutic practice that promotes emotional well-being and resilience.

A Path to Emotional Well-Being

Pregnancy emotions can be as unpredictable as a summer storm, but your journal becomes your umbrella—a source of comfort and shelter. Writing in your journal allows you to release the weight of your feelings and make space for a sense of emotional well-being.

By acknowledging and embracing your emotions, you're nurturing your emotional health. Your journal becomes a valuable tool for self-reflection, self-care, and self-compassion. It's a path to inner peace and resilience as you navigate the uncharted waters of pregnancy.

In conclusion, expressing emotions in your pregnancy journal is like embarking on an emotional journey—a way of embracing the rollercoaster of feelings that pregnancy brings. So, let your journal be your confidant, your therapist, and your cheerleader. Pour your heart onto its pages, celebrate the highs, and find solace in its embrace during the lows. Your journal is your emotional canvas, waiting for you to paint the masterpiece of your pregnancy journey—one emotion at a time.

9

Mindful Birth Preparation

As the big day approaches, mindfulness can be a valuable tool for preparing mentally and emotionally for labor and delivery.

Visualization: Use guided visualization exercises to create a mental image of a positive and empowering birth experience. Picture yourself in a serene and supportive environment, surrounded by loved ones. This mental preparation can reduce fear and increase confidence.

Visualization will become your trusted ally—a tool for reducing fear, boosting confidence, and paving the way for a positive birthing experience. Visualize your baby in your arms, on your chest, or wherever makes you feel comfortable and confident. Next, visualize you and your baby going through the birth, knowing what to do and when, trusting your instincts and your body.

The Power of Mental Preparation

Birth is a remarkable journey, and like any journey, preparation is key. Visualization is your passport to mental preparation, a way of priming your mind for a positive and empowering experience. It's like rehearsing for a grand performance, where you're the star of the show.

By mentally walking through the birthing process, you're not just reducing fear; you're also boosting your confidence. Visualization allows you to picture yourself as the resilient, strong, and courageous momma you are. It's a practice that reminds you of your innate ability to bring new life into the world.

Reducing Fear Through Visualization

As you visualize, you're also reprogramming your mind to associate birth with positivity and strength. It's like flipping the script on fear and replacing it with courage. Visualization is a way of saying to yourself, "I am ready, I am capable, and I am embracing this journey with open arms."

Keep in mind the importance of visualization, it is a way of preparing your mind and heart for a positive and empowering birth experience. Paint the picture of confidence, courage, and serenity in your mind's eye, and step into the birthing room with a heart brimming with belief in your incredible ability to bring new life into the world. Visualization is your superpower!

Mindful Acceptance: Embrace mindfulness as a way to accept and surrender to the natural process of childbirth. Recognize that birth is a transformative journey, and you have the inner strength to navigate it with mindfulness, presence, and resilience.

As you approach the transformative journey of birth, mindful acceptance becomes another one of your steadfast companions—a practice that allows you to surrender to the flow of birth with grace and resilience.

The Power of Mindful Acceptance

Childbirth is a transformative experience—a journey of profound change and growth. Mindful acceptance is your guiding philosophy, reminding you that birth, like life itself, is a natural and unpredictable process. It's like stepping onto a path with a heart full of trust, knowing that you possess the inner strength to navigate it.

Through mindfulness, you're cultivating the art of being fully present in the moment. You're letting go of resistance and allowing yourself to embrace the unfolding journey. It's like riding the waves of birth with an open heart, recognizing that each surge brings you closer to the miracle of meeting your baby.

Surrendering to the Flow

Childbirth is a river of experiences —some gentle, some intense, and all uniquely your own. As you practice mindfulness, you're surrendering to the flow of the river. You're embracing each moment with open arms, allowing it to unfold as it will. Mindful acceptance is a way of saying, "I trust in my body's ability to bring life into the world, and I surrender to the beauty of this transformative journey."

Mindful acceptance is a crucial element in preparing for childbirth, it promotes emotional well-being, enhances decision-making, and equips you with the resilience and coping skills needed for a positive birth experience. It allows you to embrace the uniqueness of your journey while reducing stress and anxiety associated with fear of the unknown.

10

Mindful Birth Plan

Being mindful can help you craft a birth plan that aligns with your values and desires while remaining flexible to the unpredictable nature of childbirth.

Research and Educate Yourself: Begin by researching different birthing options, interventions, and practices. Attend childbirth education classes and speak with your healthcare provider to understand your choices. This knowledge will empower you to make informed decisions and create a birth plan that reflects your preferences.

Birth is like a book, with each page holding a different story. Research and education allow you to read between the lines, understand the plot twists, and make informed choices. While research and creating your birth plan can be serious and thorough, it's also about finding the balance between knowledge and intuition.

The Power of Informed Decision-Making

Crafting a birth plan is like designing a blueprint for one of life's most profound experiences. Research and education are your tools, enabling you to make decisions that resonate with your heart and mind. It's like embarking on a quest, arming yourself with knowledge to navigate the twists and turns of childbirth.

By understanding different birthing options, interventions, and practices, you're not just checking boxes; you're shaping your birth experience. Knowledge empowers you to ask questions, seek alternatives, and make choices that align with your values. It's like holding a compass that points you toward a birth plan that feels authentically yours.

Creating a Flexible Birth Plan

In the realm of childbirth, flexibility is your greatest ally. Research and education allow you to create a birth plan that's not rigid but adaptable—a plan that acknowledges the unpredictable nature of childbirth. It's like writing your script with room for improvisation, knowing that sometimes the most beautiful moments are unscripted.

Dive into the world of childbirth options, interventions, and practices, and let your knowledge guide you in crafting a birth plan that reflects your heart's desires and embraces the beautiful unpredictability of childbirth.

Prioritize Your Preferences: Identify the aspects of your childbirth experience that matter most to you. Do you have a preference for certain birthing positions, pain management techniques, or who will be present during labor? Prioritize these preferences in your birth plan to ensure they are communicated clearly to your healthcare team.

Birth is like a grand adventure, filled with twists and turns. Prioritization serves as your compass, directing you toward what matters most. Let each kick be a reminder that while birth planning is a serious endeavor, it's also an opportunity to infuse your unique personality and humor into the process.

The Power of Prioritization

Childbirth is like a canvas, and prioritization is the paintbrush that allows you to bring your masterpiece to life. It's the art of selecting the colors that represent your unique vision. By identifying your priorities, you're taking charge of your birth plan's narrative. It's like being the director of your favorite movie, where every scene aligns with your heart's desires.

Prioritization empowers you to communicate clearly with your healthcare team, ensuring that your top preferences are understood and respected. It's like writing your own script for the grand performance of childbirth, where you are both the playwright and the star.

Crafting a Birth Experience That Reflects You

Childbirth is a profoundly personal journey, and your birth plan should be an equally personal reflection of your desires. Prioritization allows you to tailor your birth experience to align with your values. It's like designing a bespoke gown, meticulously crafted to fit you perfectly.

You will ultimately craft a birth plan that honors your unique wishes and ensures your top priorities shine. Dive into the world of your desires, whether it involves birthing positions, pain management techniques, or your dream support team, and prioritize them with intention and a smile. Prioritization is your spotlight, and your wishes take center stage—one priority at a time.

Use Inclusive Language: Frame your birth plan using inclusive language that emphasizes collaboration with your healthcare team. Instead of demanding specific procedures, express your preferences as wishes or desires. This approach encourages open communication and flexibility while ensuring your values are respected.

As you craft your birth plan, inclusive language becomes your bridge—a means to foster collaboration, understanding, and respect.

The Power of Words

Words have the power to create bridges or barriers. Birth planning is an opportunity to build bridges that connect you with your healthcare team. Instead of issuing commands, inclusive language invites collaboration. It's like extending a hand for a handshake, rather than pointing a finger.

By expressing your preferences as wishes and desires, you communicate your values without imposing strict demands. This approach ensures that your healthcare team understands your desires and can work with you to make informed decisions during the birthing process. It's like a symphony where every instrument plays in harmony.

Fostering Open Communication

Inclusive language opens the door to open communication. It encourages a dialogue where you, your partner, and your healthcare team can discuss options, share insights, and make decisions together. It's like sitting around a table, where everyone's voice is heard and respected.

Plan for Contingencies: Recognize that childbirth can be unpredictable, and plans may need to change. Include alternative options or contingencies in your birth plan, so you're prepared for unexpected circumstances. For example, if you initially prefer a natural birth but are open to pain relief if necessary, mention this in your plan.

Birth planning is like preparing for a grand adventure, and contingencies are your safety net, ensuring you're equipped to handle the unexpected. As you craft your birth plan, flexibility becomes one of your guiding stars—an approach to ensure you're ready for the unexpected.

Embracing the Unpredictable

Childbirth is like a story waiting to be written, but the plot can sometimes take surprising twists. Contingencies in your birth plan are like bookmarked pages, ready for exploration when the unexpected arises. It's like having an alternate ending to your favorite book, just in case.

By including alternative options or contingencies, you're acknowledging the unpredictability of childbirth while remaining adaptable. This approach ensures that you and your healthcare team are on the same page when navigating unexpected circumstances. It's like being part of a dynamic team, where everyone is ready to adjust their game plan as needed.

Fostering Peace of Mind

Contingencies provide a sense of security and peace of mind. They allow you to embrace the journey of childbirth with confidence, knowing that you're prepared for various scenarios. It's like having a well-packed suitcase for a trip —you're ready for whatever the weather or circumstances may bring.

In conclusion, preparing for contingencies in your pregnancy journal is like embarking on a quest—a way to craft a birth plan that embraces the unpredictable while maintaining flexibility and readiness. So, let your journal be your crystal ball, your alternate storyline, and your safety net. Dive into the world of contingencies, and express your openness to change and adaptability. Contingencies are your compass, and your journal is where you chart the course—one contingency at a time.

Here are some example birth plan contingencies or alternative preferences that you can include to maintain a sense of mindfulness and adaptability during labor and delivery:

   1. **Labor Environment:**

o Contingency: If the original birthing
environment is not available or suitable (e.g.,
birthing pool is occupied), I prefer an
alternative quiet and dimly lit room.

2. **Pain Management:**

o Contingency: If my chosen pain management
technique (e.g., birthing ball, breathing
exercises) is not effective, I am open to
exploring alternative comfort measures with
my birthing team.

3. **Interventions:**

o Contingency: If interventions become
medically necessary, I would like a clear
explanation from my healthcare provider
regarding the reasons and potential
alternatives.

4. **C-Section:**

o Contingency: If a cesarean section is necessary,
I request that my birthing partner be present if
possible, and I would like to have immediate
skin-to-skin contact with my baby in the
operating room.

5. **Delayed Cord Clamping:**

o

Contingency: If immediate cord clamping is necessary due to medical reasons, I request that my baby receive any available benefits of delayed cord clamping via a "cord milking" procedure.

6. **Episiotomy:**

- ○ Contingency: If an episiotomy is considered, I prefer an alternative approach, such as perineal massage or warm compresses, unless it is medically necessary.

7. **Newborn Procedures:**

- ○ Contingency: If immediate newborn assessments or procedures are required, I request that these be performed in my presence or in the same room, whenever possible, to allow for bonding and breastfeeding.

8. **Feeding Preferences:**

- ○ Contingency: If breastfeeding is not immediately possible, I would like to begin hand-expression of colostrum and receive support from a lactation consultant as soon as possible.

9. **Baby Care and Rooming-In:**

- ○

Contingency: If my baby requires medical care in the neonatal unit, I would like to be involved in their care as much as possible and receive regular updates on their condition.

10. **Emergency Contacts:**

- Contingency: If I am unable to communicate or make decisions, I designate my birth partner as my advocate and decision-maker, with the authority to consult with medical professionals on my behalf.

11. **Photography and Video:**

- Contingency: I would like my birth partner to document the birth with photos or video, but I understand that this may be limited due to medical circumstances.

12. **Visitors and Support:**

- Contingency: If my labor is prolonged or requires additional medical attention, I may need to limit the number of visitors or postpone visits until after birth.

Including these contingencies in your mindful birth plan helps you maintain a sense of mindfulness and adaptability during labor and delivery. It shows your willingness to collaborate with your healthcare team and make informed decisions while staying open to different possibilities that may arise during the birthing process.

Stay Open-Minded and Flexible: Keep in mind that childbirth is a dynamic process, and unexpected situations may arise. Cultivate a mindset of flexibility and trust in your healthcare team. Remember that the ultimate goal is a safe and healthy delivery for you and your baby. Your ability to adapt to changing circumstances is a valuable aspect of your birth plan.

Childbirth is like a dance, and you're learning the steps as you go. Staying open-minded and flexible is like being a skilled dancer, able to sway and adjust to the rhythm of the music. You trust your body and your healthcare team to lead the way.

By maintaining a mindset of flexibility, you acknowledge that childbirth is a dynamic process, and unexpected situations may arise. This approach allows you to adapt to changing circumstances with grace and trust. It's like navigating a river, where you're in the same boat as your healthcare team, rowing together toward the same goal.

The Ultimate Goal: Safe and Healthy Delivery

Above all else, the ultimate goal of childbirth is a safe and healthy delivery for you and your baby. Staying open-minded and flexible is a way to keep this goal in sight. It's like having a North Star to guide you through the darkest night—a constant reminder of what truly matters.

Pregnancy is an awe-inspiring journey—a period of profound growth, both within you and around you. Through mindfulness, you can savor every moment, from the first fluttering kicks to the peaceful stillness of waiting for your baby's arrival. As you embark on this incredible adventure, remember that you're not alone; mindfulness will be your steady companion, guiding you through the transformation of pregnancy with grace and gratitude.

11

Reflection

Pregnancy is a lot like weaving a tapestry. Each day, you add a new thread, each week, a different color, and the pattern becomes more intricate with each trimester. The art of mindful pregnancy is about stepping back to appreciate the ever-evolving design of your journey. It's about acknowledging that not every thread will be perfectly straight, and not every color will match your vision, but the final masterpiece is uniquely yours.

Remember those early days when morning sickness had you racing to the bathroom at the drop of a hat? Or those sweet moments when you first felt your baby's kicks, like a secret code between the two of you? Embrace the entire spectrum of your pregnancy experience—the good, the challenging, and the downright bizarre. These moments, whether they made you laugh, cry, or both simultaneously, are the threads that have woven your pregnancy story.

The Art of Letting Go

Throughout your mindful pregnancy journey, you've learned to let go of expectations, fears, and the need for control. Now, as you inch closer to the finish line, it's time to apply this principle one more time.

Let go of the fear of childbirth. Yes, it's natural to have butterflies in your stomach as the big day approaches, but remember that your body is designed for this. Trust in yourself and your medical team, and know that you're about to embark on one of the most profound and awe-inspiring adventures of your life.

Let go of perfection. There will be moments when you feel like you should be doing more, eating better, or preparing your baby's nursery like it's the cover of a magazine. But take a deep breath and understand that your love and presence are what truly matter. Your baby doesn't need perfection; they need you.

Let go of comparing yourself to others. Every pregnancy is unique, just like every person. Resist the urge to play the comparison game with your friends, celebrities, or the well-curated images on social media. Your journey is your own, and it's beautiful in its own way.

The Power of Presence

As you've discovered throughout your mindful pregnancy, the magic of the present moment is undeniable. Now, as you approach the final weeks, it's even more critical to tap into the power of presence. Your body is going through remarkable changes, and your baby is growing with astonishing speed. Don't miss out on these precious moments by dwelling on the past or worrying about the future.

Take the time to savor the sensations. Feel the weight of your baby bump as you cradle it in your hands. Listen to your baby's heartbeat during your prenatal check-ups, a rhythmic reminder of the life growing inside you. Cherish the hiccups, the wiggles, and those moments when your baby seems to be communicating with you in their own special language.

The Village of Support

Throughout your mindful pregnancy, you've hopefully cultivated a strong support network of family, friends, and healthcare providers. As you prepare to welcome your little one, remember that you don't have to go it alone. The village that surrounds you is there to provide the love, encouragement, and practical assistance you'll need as you transition into motherhood.

Lean on your partner for emotional support and share in the excitement and anticipation of becoming parents together. Rely on friends who have traveled this path before you, seeking their wisdom and camaraderie. Trust your healthcare team to provide guidance and expertise, and don't hesitate to ask questions or voice concerns.

The First Breath of Motherhood

The moment you hold your baby for the first time is unlike any other. It's a breathtaking experience that defies words —a surge of love, joy, and overwhelming wonder. In that moment, you officially become a mother, and it's a role that will shape the rest of your life.

As you embrace the first breath of motherhood, remember to be gentle with yourself. You're learning as you go, and that's perfectly okay. You'll have sleepless nights, messy diapers, and moments of self-doubt, but you'll also have an abundance of love, cuddles, and laughter.

Conclusion: A Mindful Motherhood

In closing, I want to express my deepest congratulations on your mindful pregnancy journey. You've nurtured not only your growing baby but also your own inner wisdom and strength. As you turn the final page of this book and embark on the incredible adventure of motherhood, remember these parting words:

Be mindful of your love. Let it flow freely and abundantly to your baby, your partner, and yourself. Love is the thread that will forever weave the tapestry of your family.

Be mindful of your patience. Motherhood is a marathon, not a sprint. Give yourself the time and space to grow and evolve as a parent.

Be mindful of your presence. Cherish every moment with your baby, for they grow all too quickly. Put down the phone, ignore the laundry, and revel in the miracle of life unfolding before your eyes.

Be mindful of your community. Lean on your village for support, and never hesitate to ask for help when you need it. You're not alone on this journey.

And finally, **be mindful of your inner strength.** You are stronger than you can imagine, and you have the capacity to navigate the challenges and joys of motherhood with grace and resilience.

As you close this book on mindful pregnancy and step into
the next chapter of your life, may your days be filled with
love, laughter, and the gentle hum of contentment.
Congratulations, dear reader, on the beautiful journey
you've embraced. Your mindful pregnancy was just the
beginning, and the adventure ahead is filled with endless
possibilities and immeasurable love.

Welcome to the extraordinary world of motherhood.

Bibliography

Aalami, M., Jafarnejad, F., & ModarresGharavi, M. (2016). The effects of progressive muscular relaxation and breathing control technique on blood pressure during pregnancy. *Iranian Journal of Nursing and Midwifery Research, 21*(3), 331. https://doi.org/10.4103/1735-9066.180382

Aşcı, Ö., & Rathfisch, G. (2016). Effect of lifestyle interventions of pregnant women on their dietary habits, lifestyle behaviors, and weight gain: a randomized controlled trial. *Journal of Health Population and Nutrition, 35*(1). https://doi.org/10.1186/s41043-016-0044-2

Beddoe, A. E., Yang, C. P., Kennedy, H. P., Weiss, S. J., & Lee, K. A. (2009). The effects of Mindfulness-Based yoga during Pregnancy on maternal psychological and physical distress. *Journal of Obstetric, Gynecologic & Neonatal Nursing, 38*(3), 310–319. https://doi.org/10.1111/j.1552-6909.2009.01023.x

Chuntharapat, S., Petpichetchian, W., & Hatthakit, U. (2008). Yoga during pregnancy: Effects on maternal comfort, labor pain and birth outcomes. *Complementary Therapies in Clinical Practice, 14*(2), 105–115. https://doi.org/10.1016/j.ctcp.2007.12.007

Duncan, L. G., & Bardacke, N. (2009). Mindfulness-Based Childbirth and Parenting Education: Promoting family mindfulness during the perinatal period. *Journal of Child and Family Studies, 19*(2), 190–202. https://doi.org/10.1007/s10826-009-9313-7

Ewy, R., & Ewy, D. (1982). *Preparation for childbirth.* Signet Book.

Fredrickson, B. L., Cohn, M., Coffey, K. A., Pek, J., & Finkel, S. M. (2008). Open hearts build lives: Positive emotions, induced through loving-kindness meditation, build consequential personal resources. *Journal of Personality and Social Psychology, 95*(5), 1045–1062. https://doi.org/10.1037/a0013262

Güder, D. S. (2018). Pregnancy Pilates and Benefits of Pregnancy Pilates during Childbirth. *Journal of Yoga and Physiotherapy, 5*(1). https://doi.org/10.19080/jyp.2018.05.555652

Haddad, E., Sabaté, J., & Whitten, C. (1999). Vegetarian food guide pyramid: a conceptual framework. *The American Journal of Clinical Nutrition, 70*(3), 615S-619S. https://doi.org/10.1093/ajcn/70.3.615s

Jallo, N., Bourguignon, C., Taylor, A. G., & Utz, S. W. (2008). Stress management during pregnancy. *Family & Community Health, 31*(3), 190–203. https://doi.org/10.1097/01.fch.0000324476.48083.41

Jerath, R., & Barnes, V. A. (2009). Augmentation of mind-body therapy and role of deep slow breathing. *Journal of*

Complementary and Integrative Medicine, 6(1).
https://doi.org/10.2202/1553-3840.1299

Lothian, J. A. (2006). Birth plans: the good, the bad, and the future. *Journal of Obstetric, Gynecologic & Neonatal Nursing,* *35*(2), 295–303. https://doi.org/10.1111/j.1552-6909.2006.00042.x

Montagu, A. (1971). *Touching: the human significance of the skin.* https://ci.nii.ac.jp/naid/10007744975/

Partanen, E., Kujala, T., Näätänen, R., Liitola, A., Sambeth, A., & Huotilainen, M. (2013). Learning-induced neural plasticity of speech processing before birth. *Proceedings of the National Academy of Sciences of the United States of America,* *110*(37), 15145–15150.
https://doi.org/10.1073/pnas.1302159110

Pino, O., Di Pietro, S., & Poli, D. (2023). Effect of Musical Stimulation on placental programming and neurodevelopment Outcome of Preterm Infants: a Systematic review. *International Journal of Environmental Research and Public Health, 20*(3), 2718.
https://doi.org/10.3390/ijerph20032718

Price, B. B., Amini, S. B., & Kappeler, K. (2012). Exercise in pregnancy. *Medicine and Science in Sports and Exercise,* 44(12), 2263–2269. https://doi.org/10.1249/mss.0b013e318267ad67

Sanders, S. (2008). Dancing through Pregnancy: Activity Guidelines for Professional and Recreational Dancers. *Journal of Dance Medicine & Science : Official Publication of the*

International Association for Dance Medicine & Science, 12(1), 17–22. https://doi.org/10.1177/1089313x0801200103

Sibley, L., Ruhling, R. O., Cameron-Foster, J., Christensen, C. L., & Bolen, T. (1981). Swimming and physical fitness during pregnancy. *Bulletin of the American College of Nurse-Midwifery, 26*(6), 3–12. https://doi.org/10.1016/0091-2182(81)90169-5

Thornton, P. L., Kieffer, E. C., Salabarría-Peña, Y., Odoms-Young, A., Willis, S. K., Kim, H., & Salinas, M. a. F. (2006). Weight, Diet, and Physical Activity-Related Beliefs and Practices among Pregnant and Postpartum Latino Women: The role of Social Support. *Maternal and Child Health Journal, 10*(1), 95–104. https://doi.org/10.1007/s10995-005-0025-3

www.ingramcontent.com/pod-product-compliance
Lightning Source LLC
Chambersburg PA
CBHW050928260726
48660CB00001B/462